THE APPLE CIDER VINEGAR MIRACLE

Harnessing the Power of Nature's Healing Elixir for Weight Loss, Digestive Health, Inflammation, Skin Care, and Radiant Vitality

By

Sharon G. Brown

TABLE OF CONTENT

Unlock the wholesome potential of Apple Cider Vinegar, which includes its health advantages, culinary uses, and practical applications. "The Apple Cider Vinegar Miracle" is the definitive resource for harnessing the potential of this time-honored treatment to achieve the highest possible level of health and energy.

Discover the many health advantages of apple cider vinegar, you will learn that it can help with digestion, promote weight loss, increase immunity, and improve skin health. With the help of straightforward recipes and do-it-yourself remedies, you can learn how to make and include apple cider vinegar into your daily routine, which will leave you feeling revitalized and invigorated.

Explore the science that underpins the healing effects of apple cider vinegar (ACV) and acquire a more in-depth understanding of how this natural tonic can assist you in achieving your health objectives. ACV has a plethora of benefits that can improve your general well-being, including the ability to maintain a healthy balance of blood sugar levels and to support the health of the heart. Whether you want to improve your health, boost your beauty regimen, or add a gourmet twist to your meals,

"The Apple Cider Vinegar Miracle " has you covered in all of these areas and more. In order to enjoy the life-changing effects of this multipurpose elixir, you should equip yourself with the information and equipment necessary to make apple cider vinegar a regular part of your routine.

CHAPTER ONE

The History and Origins of ACV

Apple cider vinegar (ACV) has a lengthy historical lineage that spans several millennia, originating from ancient civilizations like Babylonia, Egypt, Greece, and Rome. The use of vinegar for several functions, such as culinary, sanitation, and therapeutic applications, may be traced back to these ancient civilizations. The precise origins of ACV are rather ambiguous, but it is hypothesized to have derived from the process of fermenting apple juice. Apples have been grown for millennia, and their juice undergoes spontaneous fermentation upon exposure to air, resulting in the production of vinegar. Yeast is added to apple juice to accelerate the fermentation process, which converts the carbohydrates in the juice into alcohol and subsequently into acetic acid, the primary active component in vinegar.

Traditionally, apple cider vinegar (ACV) has been utilized for its therapeutic advantages and as an organic treatment for diverse illnesses. Hippocrates, an ancient Greek physician generally hailed as the "father of medicine," reportedly utilized vinegar for its medical benefits.

Vinegar has been employed historically as an antibacterial, a digestive aid, and a cure for various diseases.

Vinegar is a sour liquid produced through the fermentation process of weak alcoholic liquids, resulting in a liquid that contains acetic acid. Vinegar can be derived from several sources, such as apples or grapes (resulting in wine or cider vinegar), malted barley or oats (producing malt vinegar), and industrial alcohol (yielding distilled white vinegar). In addition, vinegars can be produced from beer, sugars, rice, and various other substances. However, vinegar likely originated as a commercial product derived from wine. Vinegar can be produced from any liquid that can undergo a two-step process to transform it into alcohol. The presence of sugar in the fruit juice or other liquid undergoes conversion into alcohol and carbon dioxide gas through the enzymatic activity of yeast. The alcohol produced in this process reacts with ambient oxygen through the activity of Acetobacter bacteria, resulting in the formation of acetic acid and water. Vinegar contains organic acids and esters that are derived from the fruit or other source material.

These compounds are responsible for the variances in flavor and scent of vinegar.

The primary purposes of vinegar are to enhance the taste of food and to preserve or pickle various types of meat, fish, fruit, and vegetables. Vinegar is frequently infused with garlic, onions, tarragon, or other herbs and spices to enhance its flavor when used as a condiment. When combined with oil and seasonings, it transforms into a traditional chilled sauce known as vinaigrette. This sauce is commonly used as a dressing for vegetable salads and as a condiment for cold cooked vegetables, meats, and fish. Vinegar is a prevalent component in marinades and is extensively employed in the pickling process of cucumbers and other vegetables.

Ancient Civilizations: Vinegar has a long history that stretches back to ancient civilizations like Babylon, Egypt, and Greece. During those times, it was commonly produced by fermenting fruit juices. Vinegar had various uses in ancient civilizations. The Babylonians employed it as a preservative and condiment, while the Egyptians utilized it for medicinal purposes and embalming.

Hippocrates and Ancient Greece:
The Greek physician Hippocrates, often referred to as the "father of modern medicine," is believed to have prescribed a mixture of honey and vinegar, similar to ACV, for various health ailments. In ancient Greece, vinegar served multiple purposes, including being used as a cleansing agent and for food preparation.

The Roman Empire: Vinegar was highly regarded by the Romans for its medicinal properties and served various purposes such as disinfection, preservation, and enhancing flavors. According to reports, Roman legionnaires consumed a concoction of vinegar and water as a tonic.

Medieval Europe: In medieval Europe, vinegar remained a valuable resource for preserving food, disinfecting wounds, and addressing different illnesses. Monks and herbalists frequently incorporated vinegar-based remedies into their practices.

Colonial America: European settlers introduced vinegar-making techniques to the New World. As a result, apple cider vinegar gained significant popularity, thanks to the abundance of apples in the region. It had multiple uses, including culinary applications and as a traditional remedy for different health issues.

In the 19th century, vinegar gained popularity as a common household item due to the publication of various books and articles highlighting its numerous health advantages. In 1820, Friedrich Mohr, a German scientist, devised a technique to measure the acidity of vinegar. This breakthrough significantly enhanced the standards of quality control in vinegar manufacturing.

In the 20th century, the popularity of ACV continued to increase as more and more individuals acknowledged its numerous health benefits. Today, apple cider vinegar continues to be widely used as a natural remedy and household product, with numerous individuals integrating it into their daily routines due to its potential health benefits.

The origins of ACV may be ancient and somewhat mysterious, but its history is a testament to its enduring popularity and perceived health benefits throughout different cultures and time periods.

CHAPTER TWO

Nutritional Composition of ACV

Recognized for its robust, sour flavor and pungent aroma, apple cider vinegar (ACV) is produced by fermenting apple juice. It is also recognized for its fermented apple juice. Despite the fact that it is mostly made up of water, apple cider vinegar (ACV) also contains a wide range of nutrients and bioactive chemicals, all of which contribute to the potential health benefits that it offers. Take a look at the following for a comprehensive breakdown of the nutritional profile of apple cider vinegar:

Acetic Acid: Apple cider vinegar is well-known for the high amount of acetic acid that it contains, which is responsible for its distinctively sour flavor and pungent odor. Acetic acid is a type of short-chain fatty acid that is created during the fermentation process. It is believed that acetic acid is responsible for many of the wellness advantages that are linked with apple cider vinegar (ACV).

Water: As is the case with the majority of liquids, apple cider vinegar is mostly made up of water, which accounts for the majority of its volume.

Vitamins: Vitamin C and a few B vitamins, such as thiamine, riboflavin, and vitamin B6 are among the vitamins that are found in apple cider vinegar (ACV), which is found in trace amounts. Despite the fact that these vitamins are only found in reasonably low amounts, they still make a contribution to the total nutritional profile of apple cider vinegar.

Minerals: Apple cider vinegar (ACV) includes trace amounts of minerals. Minerals like these are essential components in a wide variety of physiological activities that occur within the body.

Polyphenols: Apple cider vinegar (ACV) includes polyphenols, which are antioxidants that assist in protecting the body against oxidative stress and inflammation respectively. The presence of polyphenols in a wide variety of plant-based diets is thought to be a contributing factor to the health benefits of these foods.

Amino Acids: A few amino acids, which are the fundamental components of proteins, can be found in apple cider vinegar. Additionally, apple cider vinegar does contain trace levels of amino acids such as histidine, lysine, and arginine, despite the fact that it is not a significant source of protein.

Additional Bioactive Compounds: Apple cider vinegar (ACV) is a source of additional bioactive compounds, including pectin, which is a form of soluble fiber, and malic acid, which is responsible for the vinegar's sour flavor.

The exact nutritional makeup of apple cider vinegar (ACV) can change based on a number of factors, including the type of apples that are used, the fermentation process, and whether or not the vinegar is filtered or unfiltered.

It is crucial to keep this variance in mind. Nevertheless, apple cider vinegar is a nutrient-dense food that, when consumed in moderation, has the potential to be a healthy addition to your diet.

Health Benefits of Apple Cider Vinegar

Apple cider vinegar (ACV) has long been praised for its potential health benefits. Although further research is required to fully comprehend its effects, certain studies indicate that ACV may provide numerous health advantages. Presented below are a few of the possible health advantages associated with apple cider vinegar:

- **Weight Loss:** Several studies indicate that ACV might aid in weight loss by enhancing satiety and decreasing calorie consumption. Additionally, it has the potential to assist in maintaining stable blood sugar levels, potentially contributing to effective weight management.

- **Enhanced Digestion:** ACV is thought to support better digestion by boosting the production of stomach acid. It is helpful in the process of breaking down food and absorbing nutrients.

- **Blood Sugar Control:** Research indicates that ACV has the potential to enhance insulin sensitivity and reduce blood sugar levels. This could be advantageous for individuals with diabetes or those who are susceptible to the condition.

- **Heart Health:** Several animal studies indicate that ACV may have potential benefits in reducing cholesterol and triglyceride levels, both of which are associated with an increased risk of heart disease. Further investigation is required to validate these effects in human subjects.

- **Antimicrobial Properties:** ACV has long been recognized for its ability to act as a natural disinfectant and preservative, thanks to its powerful antimicrobial properties. When applied topically or used as a food preservative, it has the potential to eliminate harmful bacteria and pathogens.

- **Skin Health:** ACV is often utilized as a natural solution for skin issues like acne and eczema. Further research is required to validate its effectiveness, but it has the potential to balance the skin's pH levels and alleviate inflammation.

- **Hair Health:** For those seeking to enhance the health and shine of their hair, many individuals have turned to ACV as a natural hair rinse. Removing product buildup and balancing the scalp's pH levels can be beneficial.

- **Antioxidant Properties:** ACV is rich in polyphenols, which are known for their antioxidant properties. These compounds play a crucial role in safeguarding the body against oxidative stress and the harmful effects of free radicals.

- **Anti-Inflammatory Effects:** Research indicates that ACV has the potential to alleviate inflammation in the body, offering potential benefits for individuals with conditions like arthritis and other inflammatory disorders.

- **Enhanced Nutrient Absorption:** ACV has the potential to enhance the absorption of specific nutrients, like calcium and iron, by promoting stomach acid production and facilitating digestion.

Although the potential health benefits are promising, it is crucial to acknowledge that further research is required to gain a comprehensive understanding of the effects of ACV on human health. In addition, it is important to consume ACV in moderation to avoid potential negative effects, including tooth enamel erosion and digestive problems. If you're thinking about using ACV for its health benefits, it's advisable to seek guidance from a healthcare professional beforehand.

CHAPTER THREE

Incorporating Apple Cider Vinegar into Your Diet

A pleasant and nutritious addition to your diet, apple cider vinegar (ACV) may offer possible health benefits if you choose to include it in your diet. Use apple cider vinegar in your everyday routine in the following ways:

- **Dressings for Salads:** To make a straightforward vinaigrette, combine apple cider vinegar with olive oil, mustard, honey, and other herbs. In addition to using it as a marinade for meats and vegetables, you can also drizzle it over salads.

- **Beverages:** When it comes to beverages, you can make a pleasant drink by combining one tablespoon of apple cider vinegar with water, lemon juice, and a natural sweetener such as honey or maple syrup. To give smoothies a tangy kick, you may also add apple cider vinegar.

- **Marinades:** You can use apple cider vinegar as a foundation for marinades that you make for meats, tofu, or vegetables. The vinegar's acidity contributes to the tenderization of the food and it also imparts flavor.

- **Soups and Stews:** Adding a dash of apple cider vinegar to soups, stews, and sauces is a great way to enhance the flavor of these dishes. It is possible for it to create a more complex flavor without the need for additional salt or fat.

- **Pickling:** When it comes to pickling, apple cider vinegar can serve as a foundation for pickling veggies like cucumbers, carrots, or red onions. Vinegar not only imparts a sour flavor but also assists in the preservation of the vegetables.

- **Baking:** When baking, apple cider vinegar can be used as a leavening agent. Apple cider vinegar, when mixed with baking soda, produces bubbles that assist in the rising of baked goods.

- **Dips and Sauces:** To provide a tangy flavor to dips and sauces, such as hummus, guacamole, or salsa, you can incorporate apple cider vinegar (ACV) into the mixture.

- **Morning Tonic:** Start your day off right by preparing a morning tonic by combining one tablespoon of apple cider vinegar with one cup of warm water, one teaspoon of lemon juice, and a pinch of cinnamon. Both digestion and metabolism can be boosted as a result of this treatment.

- **Alternatives to Condiments:** Apple cider vinegar can be used as an alternative to condiments such as ketchup, mustard, or mayonnaise. Without the addition of sweets or preservatives, it imparts flavor to the dish.

When introducing apple cider vinegar into your diet, it is essential to begin with a small amount and gradually raise the dosage in order to avoid any stomach troubles. It is also recommended to select unfiltered, raw apple cider vinegar that has the "mother" still intact, as this variety of vinegar contains enzymes and probiotics

that are helpful to the environment.

DIY Home Remedies and Beauty Uses

ACV, often known as apple cider vinegar, is a versatile substance that may be utilized in a variety of cosmetic treatments and do-it-yourself (DIY) home remedies. The following is a list of detailed descriptions of how apple cider vinegar can be utilized in do-it-yourself medicines and cosmetic routines:

> **Skin Toner:** The use of apple cider vinegar (ACV) as a natural toner can help decrease acne and bring the pH levels of the skin back into balance. After

combining apple cider vinegar and water in equal parts, apply the mixture to the skin with a cotton ball, and then wait a few minutes before rinsing it off. As a result of its antibacterial characteristics, apple cider vinegar can help reduce the bacteria that cause acne and prevent breakouts.

➢ **Rinse for Hair:** Apple cider vinegar can be used as a natural hair rinse to remove buildup from hair products and to bring the pH levels of the scalp back into balance. After you have shampooed your hair, blend one-part apple cider vinegar with two parts water and apply it to your hair. After leaving it on for a few minutes, make sure you properly rinse it off. This can help enhance the health of your hair and give shine to it.

➢ **Sunburn Relief:** Apple cider vinegar (ACV) has the potential to provide treatment for burnt skin. Apply the mixture to the problematic regions using a spray bottle or a cotton ball, and make sure to mix equal proportions apple cider vinegar and water.

When applied to the skin, apple cider vinegar's anti-inflammatory qualities can help reduce redness and soothe the skin.

> **Sore Throat Remedy:** As a treatment for a sore throat, gargling with a mixture of warm water and apple cider vinegar can be helpful in providing relief. In a cup of warm water, combine one to two tablespoons of apple cider vinegar. Gargle with the mixture for thirty seconds, and then spit it out. Because of its antibacterial characteristics, apple cider vinegar can be used to destroy

bacteria and relieve inflammation.

> **Foot Soak:** When used as a foot soak, apple cider vinegar can be an effective treatment for athlete's foot as well as foot odor. Soak your feet in a mixture of one-part apple cider vinegar and two parts warm water for ten to fifteen minutes. Fungi and bacteria that are responsible for foot odor and illnesses can be eliminated with the help of apple cider vinegar's antifungal qualities.

- ➢ **Domestic Cleaner:** Due to the antibacterial qualities that it possesses, apple cider vinegar can be utilized as a natural household cleaner. Prepare a spray bottle with equal parts apple cider vinegar and water, and then use it to clean surfaces such as windows, countertops, and other areas. Apple cider vinegar's acidity can assist in the breakdown of filth and debris.

- ➢ **Digestive Aid:** If you want to enhance your digestion, drinking a mixture of water and apple cider vinegar before meals can be helpful. A glass of water with one to two tablespoons of apple cider vinegar should be consumed fifteen to thirty minutes before eating. Because of its acidity, apple cider vinegar can assist increase the formation of stomach acid and aid with digestion.

When using apple cider vinegar (ACV) in beauty treatments and do-it-yourself remedies, it is essential to dilute it with water in order to prevent skin irritation or injury. Before applying apple cider vinegar to wider regions of the skin, it is important to perform a patch test first. This is because apple cider vinegar may not be appropriate for everyone.

CHAPTER FOUR

Apple Cider Vinegar for Health and Wellness

The use of apple cider vinegar (ACV) for health and wellness has been an age-old custom spanning several centuries. Advocates of this practice assert that ACV offers a diverse array of advantages. Ongoing scientific research indicates that there are potential health benefits associated with ACV, as suggested by certain studies. In this analysis, we will explore the various applications of ACV in promoting health and wellness.

Digestive Health: ACV is thought to potentially improve digestion by stimulating the production of stomach acid. Enhancing digestion and nutrient absorption can be facilitated by this intervention. Consuming a combination of water and apple cider vinegar (ACV) prior to meals has been found to potentially enhance digestion and alleviate symptoms such as bloating and indigestion.

Blood Sugar Control: According to certain studies, ACV has the potential to enhance insulin sensitivity and reduce blood sugar levels. This could be advantageous for individuals who have diabetes or are at risk of developing the condition. ACV consumption during meals or before bedtime has been suggested to potentially regulate blood sugar levels.

Weight Management: ACV is frequently promoted as a potential tool for weight management. Several studies indicate that ACV has the potential to enhance satiety and decrease caloric consumption, potentially contributing to weight loss. Further research is required to comprehensively comprehend the impact of this phenomenon on weight management.

Heart Health: ACV has the potential to positively impact heart health by potentially reducing cholesterol and triglyceride levels. The observed effects are thought to be a result of the acetic acid and antioxidants found in ACV. However, further research is required to validate these effects.

Antimicrobial Properties: The antimicrobial properties of ACV have made it a traditional natural disinfectant and preservative. Applying it topically or using it as a food preservative has the potential to effectively eliminate harmful bacteria and pathogens.

Skin and Hair Health: Apple cider vinegar (ACV) is occasionally employed as a natural solution for various skin conditions, including acne and eczema. It could potentially assist in restoring the skin's pH balance and mitigating inflammation. In addition, apple cider vinegar (ACV) has the potential to enhance hair health and luster when used as a hair rinse.

Detoxification: There is a belief that ACV has the potential to aid in detoxification by enhancing liver function and facilitating the removal of toxins from the body. Further investigation is required to substantiate these assertions.

The use of raw, unfiltered ACV with the "mother" intact is crucial for promoting health and wellness. This type of vinegar is rich in beneficial enzymes and probiotics. In order to prevent digestive issues, it is advisable to begin with small amounts and gradually increase the dosage. It is advisable to seek guidance from a healthcare professional prior to initiating a new natural remedy regimen, as is customary.

Potential Side Effects of ACV

Apple cider vinegar (ACV) is typically safe for the majority of individuals to eat when it is used in moderation; nevertheless, there are certain potential adverse effects that should be taken into consideration, particularly when it is used in large amounts or when it is not diluted. An apple cider vinegar may have the following adverse effects:

Digestive Issues: Concerns Relating to the Digestive System Consuming undiluted apple cider vinegar or eating an excessive amount of it might irritate the digestive tract, which can result in symptoms such as nausea, stomach distress, and diarrhea. Before ingesting apple cider vinegar, it is essential to consistently dilute it with water.

Tooth Enamel Erosion: Erosion of Tooth Enamel The acidity of apple cider vinegar has the potential to erode tooth enamel if it is taken in its unadulterated form or if it does not come into frequent contact with the teeth. You should always rinse your mouth with water after eating apple cider vinegar (ACV), and you should also consider using a straw to reduce the amount of contact that your teeth have with the liquid.

Low Potassium Levels: According to the findings of a number of studies, consuming an excessive amount of apple cider vinegar over an extended period of time may result in low potassium levels in the body. This can lead to muscle weakness, cramping, and an irregular heartbeat. When using apple cider vinegar, individuals who have kidney difficulties or who are on drugs that impact potassium levels should exercise caution.

Throat and Esophageal Irritation: Inflammation of the Throat and Esophagus The acidity of undiluted apple cider vinegar has the potential to cause irritation of the throat and esophagus, particularly when ingested in large quantities or if you have a stomach that is sensitive. Always dilute apple cider vinegar with water before taking it.

Skin Irritation: Skin irritation can occur when apple cider vinegar (ACV) is applied to the skin without first being diluted, particularly for individuals who have sensitive skin. Before using apple cider vinegar (ACV) topically, it is essential to always dilute it with water and perform a patch test before applying it to wider portions of the skin.

Interactions with Drugs: Apple cider vinegar has the potential to interact with a number of drugs, including insulin, diarrhea treatments, and diuretics. For the purpose of avoiding any potential drug interactions, it is important to contact with your healthcare professional before using apple cider vinegar if you are currently taking any medications.

Allergic Reactions: There is a possibility that some individuals are allergic to apple cider vinegar (ACV) or the components that are used to manufacture it. If you suffer any indications of an allergic response, such as itching, hives, or swelling, you should immediately stop using the product and seek medical care on the matter.

In order to lessen the likelihood of experiencing adverse effects, it is essential to use apple cider vinegar in moderation and to dilute it with water before drinking it or applying it topically. Immediately discontinue the use of apple cider vinegar (ACV) and seek the advice of a qualified medical practitioner if you suffer any adverse effects that are severe or persistent.

CHAPTER FIVE

Choosing the Right Apple Cider Vinegar

The selection of an appropriate apple cider vinegar (ACV) can significantly impact both its flavor profile and potential health advantages. When choosing ACV, it is important to consider the following factors:

Raw and Unfiltered: Raw and unfiltered apple cider vinegar (ACV) is characterized by the presence of the "mother," a cloudy substance that is produced naturally during the fermentation process. The presence of beneficial enzymes and probiotics in the "mother" has the potential to provide health benefits. To maximize the nutritional benefits, it is advisable to search for ACV that is specifically labeled as raw and unfiltered.

Organic: Organic ACV is derived from apples that are grown organically, ensuring that they are devoid of synthetic pesticides and chemicals. Opting for organic apple cider vinegar (ACV) guarantees protection against potentially harmful residues.

With the Mother: The mother, as previously stated, plays a crucial role in ACV by containing advantageous enzymes and probiotics. Search for apple cider vinegar (ACV) that includes the "mother" to optimize its health advantages.

Acidity: The recommended acidity level for ACV is between 5-6%. The acidity level mentioned is considered safe for consumption and is appropriate for various culinary and household applications.

Glass Bottle: ACV, being acidic, has the potential to react with specific materials, including plastic, when stored in a glass bottle. To mitigate the risk of chemical leaching, it is advisable to opt for apple cider vinegar (ACV) that is packaged in a glass bottle.

Price: The price of ACV should not be the only consideration when making a decision. However, it is important to acknowledge that higher-quality ACV may be slightly more expensive due to factors such as the production process and the use of high-quality ingredients.

When considering the use of apple cider vinegar (ACV), it is crucial to prioritize moderation. Although apple cider vinegar (ACV) has the potential to provide health benefits, excessive consumption can result in adverse effects. Begin by consuming small quantities and progressively escalate your consumption if you so choose. It is advisable to seek guidance from a healthcare professional before incorporating ACV into your daily routine, particularly if you have any pre-existing health conditions or concerns.

Combining ACV with Other Health Practices

The integration of apple cider vinegar (ACV) with other health practices has the potential to augment its effectiveness and positively impact overall well-being. Here are some strategies for incorporating ACV into a comprehensive health regimen:

1. Balanced Diet:

The addition of ACV to salads, marinades, and beverages can enhance flavor and potentially aid digestion, contributing to a balanced diet.

To enhance digestion and regulate blood sugar levels, it is recommended to consume a glass of water diluted with a tablespoon of apple cider vinegar (ACV) prior to meals.

2. Regular Exercise:

Hydration: To maintain proper hydration during workouts, it is recommended to create a homemade sports drink by combining water, apple cider vinegar (ACV), honey, and a small amount of sea salt.

ACV can be incorporated into a post-workout tonic to potentially alleviate muscle soreness and enhance the recovery process.

3. Promoting Gut Health:

To enhance gut health, it is recommended to incorporate probiotic-rich foods such as yogurt, kefir, and fermented vegetables alongside ACV.

Incorporating prebiotic foods like garlic, onions, and bananas into your diet can provide nourishment for beneficial gut bacteria.

4. Hydration:

Morning Routine: Begin your day by consuming a glass of water infused with apple cider vinegar (ACV) and lemon juice. This hydrating drink serves as a catalyst for boosting your metabolism.

It is recommended to maintain proper hydration and flush out toxins by drinking ample water throughout the day, particularly when consuming ACV.

5. Stress Management:

Relaxation: Incorporate ACV into a warm bath containing Epsom salts to create a calming soak that has the potential to alleviate stress and promote muscle relaxation.

One way to create a soothing beverage is by combining apple cider vinegar (ACV) with calming herbal teas such as chamomile or lavender.

6. Skin Care Routine:

Natural Toner: Use diluted apple cider vinegar (ACV) as a facial toner to effectively balance the skin's pH levels and potentially alleviate acne. Apply a mixture of one-part apple cider vinegar (ACV) and two parts water using a cotton ball.

DIY Masks: Incorporating apple cider vinegar (ACV) into homemade face masks, along with ingredients such as honey and oatmeal, can provide nourishment and cleansing benefits for the skin.

7. Immune Support:

Herbal Infusions: To enhance immune support, one can create a natural tonic by combining apple cider vinegar (ACV) with immune-boosting herbs such as garlic, ginger, and turmeric.

ACV Honey Drink: The ACV Honey Drink is a soothing beverage that can be made by combining ACV, honey, and warm water. It is believed to have potential benefits in preventing colds and sore throats.

8. Weight Management:

Appetite Control: Consuming a blend of apple cider vinegar (ACV) and water prior to meals can effectively manage appetite and decrease calorie consumption.

Metabolism Boost: To enhance metabolic health, it is recommended to include apple cider vinegar (ACV) in a well-rounded diet and exercise regimen.

9. Heart Health:

Healthy Fats: One way to promote heart health is by combining ACV with healthy fats such as olive oil and avocado. This combination can result in nutritious dressings that are beneficial for cardiovascular health.

Nutrient-Rich Foods: One way to enhance the nutritional value of ACV is by incorporating it into heart-healthy foods like leafy greens, nuts, and whole grains.

10. Detoxification:

Detox Drinks: One way to detoxify is by making detox drinks. These drinks can be made by combining apple cider vinegar (ACV) with water, lemon juice, cayenne pepper, and honey.

Regular Cleanse: Incorporating apple cider vinegar (ACV) into regular detox routines can help support the body's natural detoxification processes.

CHAPTER SIX

Integrating ACV with Other Health Practices

- To prevent digestive issues, it is recommended to begin with small quantities of ACV and gradually increase the dosage.

- To optimize the potential benefits, it is recommended to consistently integrate ACV into your daily routine.

- It is important to maintain proper hydration while consuming ACV in order to facilitate detoxification and avoid dehydration.

- A balanced approach to health involves incorporating ACV into a comprehensive strategy that encompasses a nutritious diet, consistent exercise, and effective stress management techniques.

By integrating apple cider vinegar (ACV) with other health practices, individuals can adopt a comprehensive approach to wellness that promotes their overall health and well-being.

Making Apple Cider Vinegar

The process of making apple cider vinegar (ACV) from scratch is a complex and fulfilling endeavor that entails the fermentation of apple juice. Here is a detailed guide on how to make apple cider vinegar (ACV) at home:

Ingredients:

- 6-8 apples, preferably organic.

- Add 2-3 tablespoons of sugar, if desired, can accelerate the fermentation process.

- Filtered water

The apparatus:

- A large glass jar or multiple smaller jars

- Cheesecloth or a clean cloth

- Rubber band

- Knife and cutting board.

Instructions:

- Completely rinse the apples.

- To prepare the apples, cut them into small pieces, ensuring to include both the cores and peels.

Create the Apple Juice:

- Incorporate the apple pieces into either a sizable jar or several smaller jars.

- Consider adding 2-3 tablespoons of sugar, if desired. This process aids in accelerating fermentation, although it may not be essential when utilizing excessively sweet apples.

- The apples should be covered with filtered water, ensuring that there is approximately one inch of space at the top of the jar.

Cover and Store

- Use cheesecloth or a clean cloth to cover the jar and fasten it with a rubber band. By allowing the mixture to breathe, it effectively prevents the infiltration of dust and insects.

- It is recommended to store the jar in a dark and warm environment (60-80°F or 15-27°C) for approximately 2-3 weeks.

Fermentation Process:

- Regularly stirring the mixture is essential to avoid mold and promote consistent fermentation.

- After a period of 2-3 weeks, the liquid should exhibit a distinct vinegar scent and a deeper, darker hue.

Strain the Liquid:

- After the fermentation process, the apple solids can be separated by straining them using a fine-mesh sieve or cheesecloth. The resulting liquid can then be transferred to a clean jar.

Secondary Fermentation:

- The jar should be covered with a cloth and allowed to sit for an additional 3-4 weeks, with occasional stirring. During the initial fermentation process, the alcohol generated will undergo a conversion into acetic acid, resulting in the liquid acquiring vinegar-like characteristics.

Taste and Store

- Taste the vinegar. Once the acidity level has been achieved, the product is deemed suitable for bottling. If not, try allowing it to ferment for a little longer.

- The ACV should be transferred to a glass bottle with a tight-fitting lid and stored once it is ready.

Tips for Long-Term Use

When used carefully and responsibly, incorporating apple cider vinegar (ACV) into your lifestyle over time can have a long-lasting positive impact on your health. Here are some pointers to guarantee the long-term, safe and efficient usage of ACV:

1. Dilution Is Crucial

Never take ACV undiluted. To avoid irritating the lining of the stomach and esophagus, combine 1-2 tablespoons of apple cider vinegar with a big glass of water (8–12 ounces).

Use in Cooking Instructions: To reap the advantages of apple cider vinegar (ACV) without running the risk of ingesting it raw, try adding it to marinades, salad dressings, and other dishes.

2. Moderation Is Essential

Follow Recommended Amounts: Don't take more than one or two tablespoons daily. Negative side effects including low potassium levels and loss of bone density might result from excessive intake.

Prevent Abuse: It's not always better to have more. Overindulgence in ACV can lead to several health problems, including intestinal distress.

3. Protect Your Teeth

Use a Straw: To decrease contact with your teeth and lower the risk of enamel erosion, drink ACV diluted with water through a straw.

Rinse Your Mouth: To assist remove any remaining acidity, rinse your mouth with plain water after taking ACV.

Wait to Brush: To prevent more erosion of the enamel, wait at least half an hour after ingesting ACV before cleaning your teeth.

4. Keep an eye on Your Body's Reaction

Pay Attention to Your Body: Observe how ACV affects your body's response. Modify your dosage if you encounter any negative side effects, such as gastrointestinal problems or skin discomfort.

Consult a Physician: Before incorporating ACV into your diet on a regular basis, speak with your healthcare practitioner if you have any pre-existing medical conditions or are taking any drugs.

5. Quality Is Important

Select the Right Type: For optimal health effects, use organic, raw, unfiltered, and "mother" ACV. Probiotics, proteins, and helpful enzymes can all be found in the "mother".

Keep Safe: To preserve its quality and increase its shelf life, store your ACV in a cold, dark area and make sure the cap is well shut.

6. Incorporate in a Well-Balanced Diet

Variety in Consumption: To keep your diet interesting and varied, use apple cider vinegar (ACV) in a range of applications, such as marinades, beverages, and even cooking.

Nutrient-Rich Diet: To enhance general health, use ACV with a diet high in fruits, vegetables, lean meats, and whole grains.

7. Combine with Other Healthy Routines

Frequent Exercise: To maximize the potential advantages of ACV on metabolism and weight management, combine your intake with frequent physical activity.

Sufficient Hydration: Stay hydrated by drinking lots of water throughout the day, especially after taking ACV, to help flush out toxins and preserve general health.

8. Use Caution When Using for Skin and Hair Care

Patch Test: To make sure you don't have any negative side effects, always do a patch test prior to applying ACV topically.

Dilution for Topical Use: To prevent irritation, dilute apple cider vinegar (ACV) with water (about 1 part ACV to 2 parts water) when using it as a toner or hair rinse.

9. Daily Routine:

Consistency is Important To optimize ACV's potential health advantages, incorporate it into your daily routine on a continuous basis.

Long-Term Commitment: Give your body time to acclimate to adding ACV to your diet by being patient. Regular, consistent use yields long-term advantages.

These pointers will help you include ACV into your long-term wellness and health regimen in a safe and efficient manner, allowing you to maximize its potential advantages and minimize its hazards.

Tips:

- The addition of a few tablespoons of raw, unfiltered apple cider vinegar with the "mother" can potentially accelerate the fermentation process.

- To prevent mold growth, it is important to clean all equipment and fully submerge the apples in the liquid.

- Patience is crucial when it comes to developing a rich and flavorful vinegar, as the fermentation process typically spans several weeks to months.

Enjoy your homemade apple cider vinegar!

END